Hepatitis A
DIET COOKBOOK
For Seniors

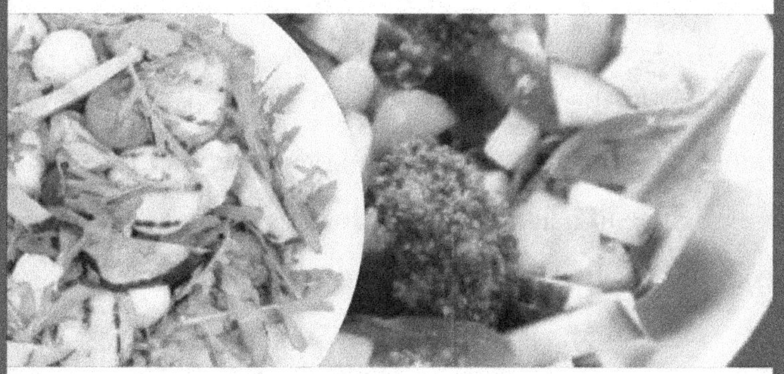

Nourishing Recipes for Liver Health, Recovery, and Enhanced Well-Being

Leona Butler

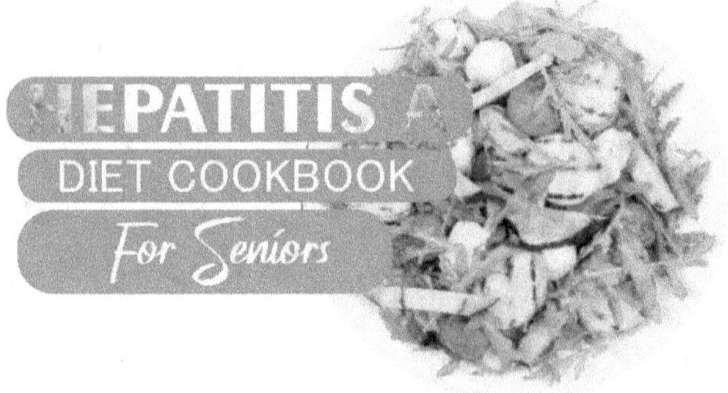
HEPATITIS A
DIET COOKBOOK
For Seniors

9 easy steps how to use a hepatitis A Diet Cookbook For Seniors

1. Get this Cookbook: Obtain a hepatitis A Diet Cookbook specifically tailored for seniors. You can find these at bookstores, online retailers, or libraries.

2. Read Introduction: Start by reading the introduction section of the cookbook. This usually contains important information about the diet plan, its benefits, and tips for success.

3. Understand Dietary Guidelines: Familiarize yourself with the dietary guidelines provided in the cookbook. These guidelines are usually designed to support liver health and prevent further complications from hepatitis A.

4. Plan Your Meals: Take some time to plan your meals for the week. Look through the recipes in the cookbook and select ones that appeal to you and fit within the dietary guidelines.

5. Grocery Shopping: Make a list of ingredients you'll need for the selected recipes and go grocery shopping. Choose fresh, whole foods that are recommended for a liver-friendly diet.

6. Meal Preparation: Follow the recipes in the cookbook to prepare your meals. Pay attention to portion sizes and cooking methods to ensure they align with the dietary recommendations.

7. Stay Hydrated: Drink plenty of water throughout the day to stay hydrated. Adequate hydration is essential for overall health and can help support liver function.

8. Monitor Your Progress: Keep track of how you feel and any changes in your health as you follow the diet plan. This will help you determine if the diet is having a positive impact on your well-being.

9. Stay Consistent: Stick to the diet plan consistently to reap its benefits. Remember that dietary changes take time to show results, so be patient and stay committed to your health goals.

4

TABLE OF CONTENT

Introduction

Welcome to the 'Hepatitis A Diet Cookbook For elders,' a complete resource designed to help elders recover from Hepatitis A. This cookbook provides numerous benefits aimed at improving the well-being of elders living with this ailment. Inside, you'll find a carefully curated variety of recipes designed to boost nutritional support, enhance liver health, and aid in the healing process. Our simple recommendations ensure that seniors can follow their dietary limitations while still enjoying flavor and variety.

This cookbook reduces problems and speeds up the recovery process by combining antioxidant-rich nutrients and liver-supportive foods. Our cookbook strives to empower seniors by providing tasty, healthy meals that encourage healing and overall well-being. Say goodbye to dull, limiting diets and hello to a journey of vibrant health with our 'Hepatitis A Diet Cookbook For Seniors.'"

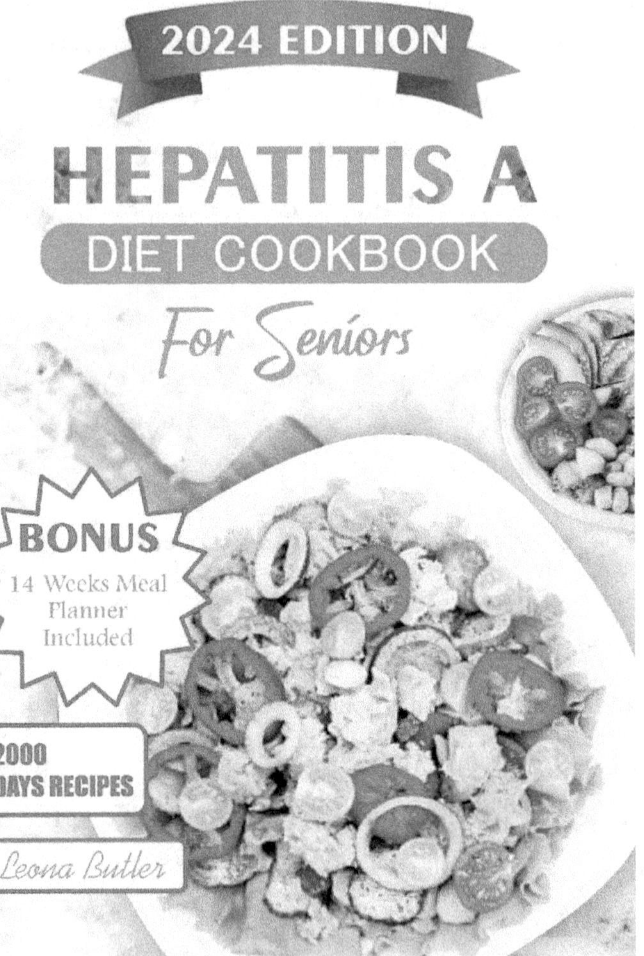

2024 EDITION
HEPATITIS A
DIET COOKBOOK
For Seniors
BONUS
14 Weeks Meal
Planner
Included
2000
DAYS RECIPES
Leona Butler

Chapter 1: Understanding Hepatitis A

Hepatitis A is a contagious liver ailment caused by the Hepatitis A virus. It is transmitted through the intake of contaminated food or water, or through personal contact with an infected individual. Hepatitis A symptoms include fatigue, nausea, stomach pain, jaundice, and black urine. While most people recover completely from Hepatitis A with no long-term liver damage, severe instances can lead to liver failure, particularly in elderly adults.

Importance of Diet in Managing Hepatitis A:

Diet is crucial in managing Hepatitis A, especially for elderly. A balanced diet can help to improve liver function, stimulate the immune system, and speed up the recovery process. Seniors with Hepatitis A should eat meals that are easy to digest, soft on the liver, and high in important nutrients. This includes:

- Lean proteins: Seniors should include poultry, fish, tofu, and beans in their diet. Protein helps to repair liver cells and promotes overall health.

- Fruits and veggies: Fresh fruits and vegetables are high in vitamins, minerals, and antioxidants, which can help liver function and reduce inflammation. Seniors should attempt to incorporate a range of colored fruits and vegetables into their diets.

- Whole grains, such as brown rice, quinoa, and oats, include fiber and important minerals that promote digestive health and maintain consistent energy levels.

- Healthy fats: Nuts, seeds, avocado, and olive oil include unsaturated fats that can help reduce inflammation and promote heart health. Seniors should restrict their intake of saturated and trans fats, which are present in processed foods and fried goods.

- Hydration: Staying hydrated is essential for liver function and general health. Seniors should drink lots of water throughout the day and restrict their intake of sugary beverages and alcohol.

Target Audience: Seniors:

This handbook is specifically designed to meet the needs of seniors who have Hepatitis A or are at risk of developing the disease. Seniors frequently encounter particular obstacles while managing health issues, and this resource strives to provide practical advice and assistance as they negotiate the complexity of Hepatitis A management.

How This Book Can Help:

This book encourages readers to take charge of their health and make informed decisions by giving detailed information on Hepatitis A and emphasizing the relevance of nutrition in controlling the condition in seniors.

Through practical ideas, nutritional recommendations, and insights into the special needs of seniors, readers will obtain the knowledge and confidence to effectively manage Hepatitis A and enhance overall well-being.

Nutritional Needs for Seniors with Hepatitis A

Hepatitis A, a viral infection that affects the liver, can be especially difficult for seniors since their immune systems may be weakened and recovery times are longer. Proper nutrition is essential for maintaining liver health and overall well-being during and after hepatitis A infection. Seniors with hepatitis A should eat a healthy diet that supports liver function, increases immunity, and promotes healing.

Foods to Avoid and Limit

- Certain foods can worsen liver inflammation and impede recovery in people with hepatitis A. Senior citizens should avoid or minimize the following:

- Fatty and fried foods can stress the liver and exacerbate inflammation. Seniors should limit their consumption of fried foods, fatty meats, and processed snacks.

- Alcohol: Alcohol can damage the liver and impair medication effectiveness. Seniors with hepatitis A should avoid alcohol altogether during their recuperation.

- Sugary foods and beverages: A high sugar intake can lead to insulin resistance and inflammation. Seniors should limit their intake of sugary snacks, desserts, and sweetened drinks.

- Salty diets: High-sodium diets can cause fluid retention and increase liver edema. Seniors should reduce their consumption of processed foods, canned soups, and salty snacks.

- Raw or Undercooked shellfish: Hepatitis A is frequently spread through infected food or water, especially raw or undercooked shellfish. Seniors should prepare all seafood properly to avoid the risk of infection.

A healthy diet can assist elders with hepatitis A manage their symptoms, support liver function, and promote recovery. Here's how to prepare a healthful food plan:

- Focus on Whole Foods: Include whole grains, fruits, vegetables, lean proteins, and healthy fats. Whole foods contain critical nutrients, antioxidants, and fiber, which promote general health.

- Include Lean Proteins: Choose lean protein sources including chicken, fish, tofu, beans, and lentils. Protein is essential for tissue regeneration and immunological function during hepatitis A healing.

- Prioritize Fruits and Vegetables: Colorful fruits and vegetables are high in vitamins, minerals, and antioxidants, which promote liver health and immunity. Aim to incorporate a variety of produce into each meal.

- Choose Healthy Fats: Include sources of healthy fats including avocados, nuts, seeds, and olive oil. These lipids contain important fatty acids, which promote cellular function and prevent inflammation.

- Stay Hydrated: Adequate hydration is essential for liver function and general health. Seniors should drink enough of water throughout the day and consume hydrating foods such as soups, smoothies, and watery fruits.

- Moderate Fiber Intake: While fiber is important for digestive health, consuming too much can cause bloating and discomfort, especially for individuals with liver inflammation. Seniors should aim for moderate fiber intake from whole grains, fruits, and vegetables.

- Limit Sodium: Reduce sodium intake to help prevent fluid retention and swelling. Choose fresh or minimally processed foods, and avoid adding extra salt to meals.

- Consider Supplements: Seniors with hepatitis A may benefit from certain supplements under the guidance of a healthcare provider, such as vitamin D, B vitamins, and omega-3 fatty acids.

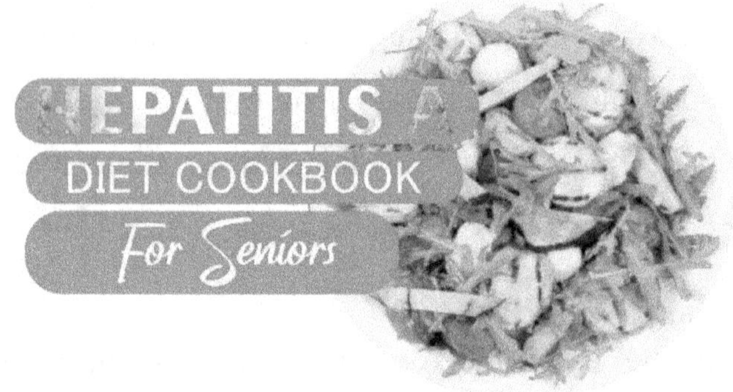

Chapter 2: Breakfast Recipes

1. Oatmeal with Blueberries:

Ingredients:

- 1/2 cup rolled oats
- 1 cup water or milk (your choice)
- 1/4 cup blueberries
- Optional toppings: honey, chopped nuts, cinnamon

Preparation:

1. In a small saucepan, heat the water or milk until it boils.
2. Stir in the rolled oats and decrease the heat to low. Cook for 5 minutes, stirring regularly, until the oats are cooked and the mixture thickens.
3. Remove from heat and let it sit for a minute.
4. Transfer the oatmeal to a bowl and top with blueberries and any other desired toppings. Serve hot.

Nutritional Value:

- Calories: Approximately 150-200 (depending on milk vs. water and toppings)
- Protein: Around 5-7 grams
- Fiber: 4-6 grams
- Healthy fats from nuts or avocado, if added

Cooking Time: 5-7 minutes

2. Scrambled Eggs with Spinach

Ingredients:

- 2 large eggs
- 1 cup fresh spinach leaves
- Salt and pepper to taste 1 tablespoon olive oil or butter

Preparation:

1. Heat olive oil or butter in a non-stick skillet over medium heat.
2. In a bowl, beat the eggs and season with salt and pepper.

3. Add the beaten eggs to the skillet and let them cook for a minute.

4. Add spinach leaves to the skillet and continue cooking, stirring gently, until the eggs are fully cooked and the spinach is wilted.

5. Remove from heat and transfer to a plate.

6. Serve hot.

Nutritional Value:

- Calories: Approximately 150-200

- Protein: Around 12-14 grams

- Vitamins and minerals from spinach

Cooking Time: 5-7 minutes

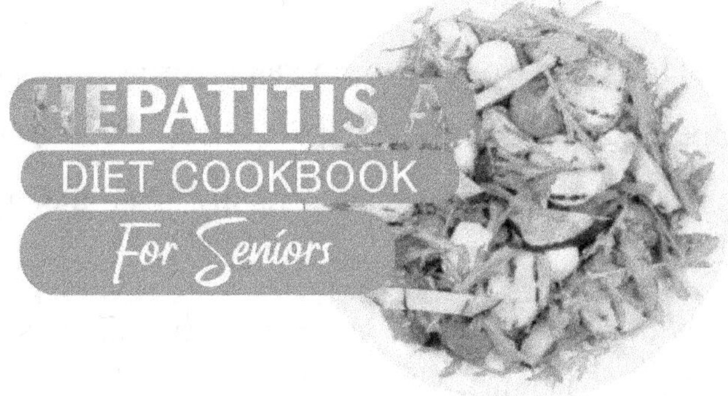

3. Whole Wheat Toast with Avocado:

Ingredients:

- 2 slices whole wheat bread
- 1 ripe avocado
- Salt and pepper to taste
- Optional toppings: red pepper flakes, sliced tomatoes, sprouts

Preparation:

1. Toast the whole wheat bread slices until golden brown.
2. While the bread is toasting, scoop out the flesh of the avocado into a bowl.
3. Use a fork to mash the avocado and season with salt and pepper.
4. Spread the mashed avocado equally over the toasted bread slices.
5. Top with any additional toppings as desired.
6. Serve immediately.

Nutritional Value:

- Calories: Approximately 200-250
- Healthy fats from avocado
- Fiber from whole wheat bread

Cooking Time: 2-3 minutes (toasting bread)

4. Greek Yogurt Parfait:

Ingredients:

- 1 cup Greek yogurt
- 1/2 cup granola
- 1/2 cup mixed berries (strawberries, blueberries, raspberries) Honey (optional, to taste)

Preparation:

1. In a serving glass or bowl, layer Greek yogurt, granola, and mixed berries.
2. Repeat layers until ingredients are used up.
3. Drizzle honey on top if desired.

Nutritional Value:

- Protein: ~20g (depends on yogurt and granola)
- Fiber: ~5g (depends on granola and berries)
- Calories: ~300-400 (depending on quantities and additions)

5. Smoothie with Spinach and Banana

Ingredients:

- 1 ripe banana
- 1 cup spinach leaves
- 1/2 cup almond milk
- 1/2 cup plain Greek yogurt 1 tablespoon honey (optional)

Preparation:

1. Place all ingredients in a blender.
2. Blend until smooth and creamy.
3. Add more almond milk if necessary to reach desired consistency.

Serve immediately.

Nutritional Value:

- Protein: ~10g

- Fiber: ~5g

- Calories: ~200-250 (depending on quantities and additions)

6. Quinoa Breakfast Bowl

Ingredients:

- 1/2 cup quinoa

- 1 cup water or milk (for cooking quinoa)

- 1 tablespoon honey or maple syrup

- 1/2 teaspoon cinnamon

- 1/4 cup chopped nuts (such as almonds, walnuts, or pecans)

- 1/4 cup dried fruits (such as raisins, cranberries, or apricots) Fresh fruit (such as sliced banana, berries, or apple)

Preparation:

1. Rinse quinoa under cold water.
2. In a saucepan, combine quinoa and water or milk. Bring to a boil.
3. Reduce the heat to low, cover, and let simmer for about 15 minutes, or until the quinoa is cooked and the liquid is absorbed.
4. Fluff quinoa with a fork and stir in honey or maple syrup and cinnamon.
5. Divide cooked quinoa into serving bowls.
6. Top with chopped nuts, dried fruits, and fresh fruit.

Nutritional Value:

- Protein: ~10g
- Fiber: ~5g
- Calories: ~300-400 (depending on quantities and additions)

Cooking Time: Approximately 20 minutes

7. Vegetable Omelette

Ingredients:

- 2 large eggs
- 1/4 cup diced bell peppers
- 1/4 cup diced tomatoes
- 1/4 cup diced onions
- 1/4 cup chopped spinach
- Salt and pepper to taste 1 tablespoon olive oil

Preparation:

1. In a bowl, beat the eggs until well combined.
2. Stir in the diced bell peppers, tomatoes, onions, and chopped spinach. Season with salt and pepper.
3. In a nonstick skillet, heat the olive oil on medium heat.
4. Pour the egg mixture into the skillet and cook for 2-3 minutes until the bottom is set.
5. Flip the omelette and cook for another 2-3 minutes until fully cooked. Serve hot, optionally garnished with fresh herbs.

Nutritional Value: This vegetable omelette is high in protein, vitamins, and minerals, providing a balanced meal option.

Cooking Time: Approximately 5-7 minutes.

8. Cottage Cheese with Pineapple:

Ingredients:

- 1 cup cottage cheese
- 1 cup diced pineapple
- Honey or maple syrup for drizzling (optional)

Preparation:

1. Place the cottage cheese in a bowl.
2. Add the diced pineapple on top.
3. Drizzle with honey or maple syrup if desired.
4. Serve chilled as a refreshing breakfast or snack option.

9. Whole Grain Pancakes:

Ingredients:

- 1 cup whole grain flour
- 1 tablespoon baking powder
- 1 tablespoon honey or maple syrup
- 1 cup milk (dairy or plant-based) 1 large egg
- 1 tablespoon melted butter or oil
- Pinch of salt

Preparation:

1. In a mixing bowl, combine the whole grain flour, baking powder, and salt.
2. In another bowl, whisk together the honey or maple syrup, milk, egg, and melted butter or oil. Pour the wet ingredients into the dry ingredients and stir just until mixed. Do not overmix the batter; it is fine if it is somewhat lumpy.
3. Heat a nonstick skillet or griddle over medium heat, then gently coat with oil or butter.

4. Pour 1/4 cup batter into the skillet for each pancake.

5. Cook until bubbles appear on the surface, then flip and cook until golden brown on the opposite side.

6. Serve hot with your favorite toppings such as fresh fruit, nuts, or yogurt.

Nutritional Value: These whole grain pancakes are a good source of fiber, protein, and essential nutrients, making them a wholesome breakfast choice.

Cooking Time: Approximately 10-15 minutes.

10. Egg and Veggie Muffins:

Ingredients:

- 6 large eggs
- 1/4 cup diced bell peppers
- 1/4 cup diced onions
- 1/4 cup chopped spinach
- Salt and pepper to taste Cooking spray or oil for greasing

Preparation:

1. Preheat the oven to 350°F (175°C). Grease a muffin tin with cooking spray or oil.
2. In a bowl, beat the eggs until well combined.
3. Stir in the diced bell peppers, onions, and chopped spinach. Season with salt and pepper. Pour the egg mixture equally into the muffin cups, filling them approximately 3/4 full. Bake in the preheated oven for 20-25 minutes, or until the egg muffins are firm and gently browned on top.
4. Remove from the oven and allow it cool for a few minutes before serving.
5. Enjoy warm or refrigerate for later consumption.

Nutritional Value: These egg and veggie muffins are a protein-rich and nutritious breakfast option, packed with vitamins and minerals from the vegetables.

Cooking Time: Approximately 20-25 minutes.

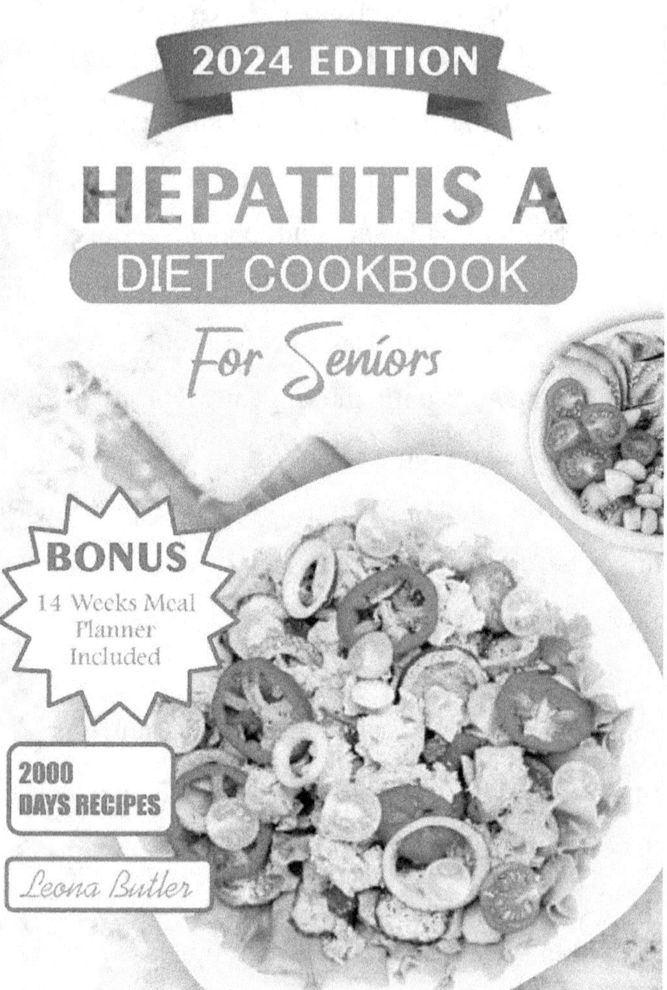

2024 EDITION
HEPATITIS A
DIET COOKBOOK
For Seniors
BONUS
14 Weeks Meal
Planner
Included
2000
DAYS RECIPES
Leona Butler

Chapter 3: Lunch recipes

1. Grilled Chicken Salad

Ingredients:

- 2 boneless, skinless chicken breasts (about 8 ounces each)
- 6 cups mixed salad greens
- 1 cup cherry tomatoes, halved
- cucumber, sliced
- 1/4 cup red onion, thinly sliced
- 1/4 cup crumbled feta cheese
- tablespoons olive oil
- 2 tablespoons balsamic vinegar Salt and pepper to taste

Preparation:

1. Preheat grill to medium-high heat.
2. Season chicken breasts with salt and pepper.
3. Grill chicken for 6-8 minutes per side, or until cooked through (internal temperature of 165°F).

4. Let the chicken rest for 5 minutes before slicing into thin pieces.

5. In a large bowl, combine salad greens, cherry tomatoes, cucumber, red onion, and feta cheese. In a small bowl, whisk together olive oil and balsamic vinegar to make the dressing. Toss salad with dressing.

6. Top salad with grilled chicken strips.

7. Serve immediately.

Nutritional Value:

- Calories: Approximately 350 per serving
- Protein: Approximately 30g per serving
- Carbohydrates: Approximately 10g per serving Fat: Approximately 20g per serving

Cooking Time:

15-20 minutes

2. Tuna Salad Wrap

Ingredients:

- can (5 ounces) tuna, drained
- tablespoons mayonnaise
- tablespoon Dijon mustard
- 1/4 cup diced celery
- 1/4 cup diced red onion
- Salt and pepper to taste
- large whole wheat tortillas
- 1 cup mixed salad greens

Preparation:

- In a mixing bowl, combine tuna, mayonnaise, Dijon mustard, celery, and red onion.
- Season with salt and pepper, to taste.
- Lay tortillas flat on a clean surface.
- Divide tuna salad mixture evenly between the two tortillas, spreading it out in the center of each.
- Top each with a handful of mixed salad greens.

- Roll the tortillas tightly and fold in the sides as you go.

- Divide each wrap in half diagonally.

- Serve immediately or store in foil for later.

Nutritional Value:

- Calories: Approximately 300 per serving

- Protein: Approximately 20g per serving

- Carbohydrates: Approximately 30g per serving Fat: Approximately 10g per serving

Cooking Time:

10 minutes

3. Vegetable Soup

Ingredients:

- 2 tablespoons olive oil

- onion, chopped

- carrots, diced

- 2 stalks celery, diced

- 2 cloves garlic, minced

- 1 can (14.5 ounces) diced tomatoes

- 4 cups vegetable broth

- 1 teaspoon dried thyme

- 1 teaspoon dried oregano

- 1 cup chopped spinach Salt and pepper to taste

Preparation:

1. In a large pot, heat the olive oil over medium heat.
2. Add the chopped onions, carrots, celery, and garlic. Cook until the vegetables are soft, about 5-7 minutes.
3. Stir in diced tomatoes, vegetable broth, thyme, and oregano.
4. Bring soup to a simmer and let it cook for 15-20 minutes.
5. Add chopped spinach and cook for an additional 5 minutes.
6. Season with salt and pepper, to taste.
7. Serve hot.

Nutritional Value:

- Calories: Approximately 120 per serving

- Protein: Approximately 3g per serving

- Carbohydrates: Approximately 15g per serving Fat: Approximately 6g per serving

Cooking Time:
30-35 minutes

4. Quinoa Salad

Ingredients:

- cup quinoa
- cups water or vegetable broth
- 1 cucumber, diced
- bell pepper, diced
- 1/4 cup red onion, finely chopped
- 1/4 cup fresh parsley, chopped
- 1/4 cup feta cheese, crumbled (optional)
- 1/4 cup olive oil
- tablespoons lemon juice Salt and pepper to taste

Preparation:

1. Rinse quinoa under cold water.
2. Heat water or vegetable broth in a pot until it boils. Add quinoa, reduce heat to low, cover, and simmer for 15-20 minutes until liquid is absorbed and quinoa is tender.
3. Remove from heat and allow to cool.
4. In a large bowl, combine cooked quinoa, diced cucumber, bell pepper, red onion, parsley, and feta cheese.
5. In a small bowl, whisk together olive oil, lemon juice, salt, and pepper. Pour over the salad and toss to combine.
6. Serve chilled or at room temperature.

Nutritional Value:

- Quinoa is high in protein, fiber, and various vitamins and minerals such as magnesium, phosphorus, and iron.
- Cucumber, bell pepper, and parsley add vitamins and minerals like vitamin C and K.
- Feta cheese provides calcium and protein. Olive oil offers healthy fats.

Cooking Time: 20-25 minutes

5. Turkey and Avocado Sandwich

Ingredients:

- 4 slices whole grain bread
- 8 slices roasted turkey breast
- 1 avocado, sliced
- 1 tomato, sliced
- 1/4 cup lettuce leaves
- Mustard or mayonnaise (optional)
- Salt and pepper to taste

Preparation:

1. Toast the bread slices if desired.
2. Put mustard or mayonnaise on one side of each bread slice.
3. Layer turkey slices, avocado slices, tomato slices, and lettuce leaves on two slices of bread.
4. Season with salt and pepper.

5. Top with the remaining bread slices.

6. Cut sandwiches in half if desired and serve.

Nutritional Value:

- Whole grain bread contains fiber and important minerals.

- Turkey breast is a lean protein source.

- Avocado offers healthy fats, fiber, and various vitamins and minerals.

- Tomato and lettuce contribute vitamins and minerals.

Cooking Time: 10 minutes

6. Salmon and Asparagus

Ingredients:

- 2 salmon fillets (about 6 oz each)

- bunch asparagus, trimmed

- tablespoons olive oil

- 2 cloves garlic, minced

- 1 lemon, sliced

- Salt and pepper to taste

- Fresh herbs (such as parsley or dill) for garnish (optional)

Preparation:

1. Preheat oven to 400°F (200°C).
2. Place salmon fillets on a baking pan lined with parchment paper.
3. Arrange the asparagus on the baking sheet, surrounding the salmon.
4. Drizzle olive oil over salmon and asparagus. Sprinkle minced garlic evenly.
5. Place lemon slices on top of the salmon fillets.
6. Season everything with salt and pepper.
7. Bake in the preheated oven for 12-15 minutes, or until salmon is cooked through and flakes easily with a fork.
8. Garnish with fresh herbs if desired and serve.

Nutritional Value:

- Salmon is rich in omega-3 fatty acids, high-quality protein, and various vitamins and minerals like vitamin D and selenium.
- Asparagus is low in calories and rich in fiber, vitamins A, C, E, and K, as well as folate.
- Olive oil provides healthy fats.

Cooking Time: 15 minutes

7. Mushroom and Spinach Quesadilla:

Ingredients:

- 2 large flour tortillas
- cup sliced mushrooms
- cups fresh spinach
- 1 cup shredded cheese (such as cheddar or mozzarella)
- Olive oil
- Salt and pepper to taste

Preparation:

1. Heat a sprinkle of olive oil in a skillet over medium heat.

2. Sauté the sliced mushrooms until they release moisture and turn golden brown, about 5-7 minutes.

3. Add fresh spinach to the skillet and cook until wilted, about 2-3 minutes.

4. Season with salt and pepper to taste.

5. Remove the mushroom and spinach mixture from the skillet and set aside.

6. Place a tortilla in the skillet and evenly distribute half of the grated cheese.

7. Spread the mushroom and spinach mixture over the cheese.

8. Sprinkle the remaining cheese over the mushroom and spinach mixture.

9. Top with the second tortilla.

10. Cook until the bottom tortilla is golden brown and crispy, about 3-4 minutes.

11. Carefully flip the quesadilla and cook until the other side is golden brown and crispy, about 2-3 minutes more.

12. Remove from the skillet and let cool for a minute before
slicing.
Serve warm.

cooking time: 15 minutes.

8. Bean and Vegetable Wrap

Ingredients

- 2 large whole wheat tortillas
- 1 can (15 oz) of black beans, drained and rinsed
- 1 cup diced bell peppers (any color)
- 1 cup diced tomatoes
- 1 cup shredded lettuce
- 1/2 cup diced red onion
- 1 avocado, sliced
- 1/4 cup salsa
- 1/4 cup Greek yogurt or sour cream Salt and pepper to taste

Preparation:

1. In a bowl, mash the black beans with a fork until slightly chunky.
2. Lay out the tortillas and spread the mashed black beans evenly over each.
3. Layer the diced bell peppers, tomatoes, shredded lettuce, diced red onion, and avocado slices over the beans.
4. Drizzle salsa and Greek yogurt or sour cream over the vegetables.
5. Season with salt and pepper to taste.
6. Roll the tortillas tightly and fold in the sides as you go.
7. Cut each wrap in half diagonally.
8. Serve immediately or cover securely in foil to store for later.

Nutritional Value: This wrap is packed with fiber, protein, vitamins, and minerals from the beans and vegetables. Approximate
cooking time: 10 minutes.

9. Egg Salad Lettuce Wraps:

Ingredients:

- 6 hard-boiled eggs, chopped 1/4 cup mayonnaise

- 2 tablespoons Dijon mustard

- 1/4 cup diced celery

- 2 tablespoons chopped fresh dill

- Salt and pepper to taste

- 6 large lettuce leaves (such as butter or romaine)

Preparation:

1. In a bowl, combine chopped hard-boiled eggs, mayonnaise, Dijon mustard, diced celery, and chopped fresh dill.
2. Mix well until evenly combined.
3. Season with salt and pepper to taste.
4. Spooning the egg salad mixture onto each lettuce leaf.
5. Roll up the lettuce leaves like a burrito, tucking in the sides as you go.

Nutritional Value: This dish is rich in protein, healthy fats, and vitamins from the eggs and vegetables. Approximate

cooking time: 15 minutes (including boiling eggs).

10. Quinoa Stuffed Bell Peppers

Ingredients:

- 4 large bell peppers (any color)
- cup quinoa, rinsed
- cups vegetable broth or water
- 1 can (15 oz) of black beans, drained and rinsed
- 1 cup corn kernels (fresh or frozen)
- cup diced tomatoes
- 1/2 cup diced red onion
- cloves garlic, minced
- 1 teaspoon cumin
- 1 teaspoon chili powder
- Salt and pepper to taste 1 cup shredded cheese (optional)

Preparation:

Preheat the oven to 375°F (190°C).

1. Remove the seeds and membranes from the bell peppers by cutting off the top.

2. In a saucepan, combine quinoa and vegetable broth or water. Bring to a boil, then reduce heat to low, cover, and simmer until quinoa is cooked and liquid is absorbed, about 15-20 minutes. In a large bowl, mix cooked quinoa, black beans, corn kernels, diced tomatoes, diced red onion, minced garlic, cumin, chili powder, salt, and pepper.

3. Spoon the quinoa mixture into each bell pepper until filled.

4. Place stuffed bell peppers in a baking dish and cover with foil.

5. Bake in a preheated oven for 25-30 minutes, or until the peppers are soft..

6. If using cheese, remove the foil during the last 5 minutes of baking and sprinkle shredded cheese over the tops of the peppers.

7. Serve hot.

Nutritional Value: These stuffed bell peppers are high in fiber, protein, vitamins, and minerals from the quinoa, black beans, and vegetables. Approximate

cooking time: 45-50 minutes.

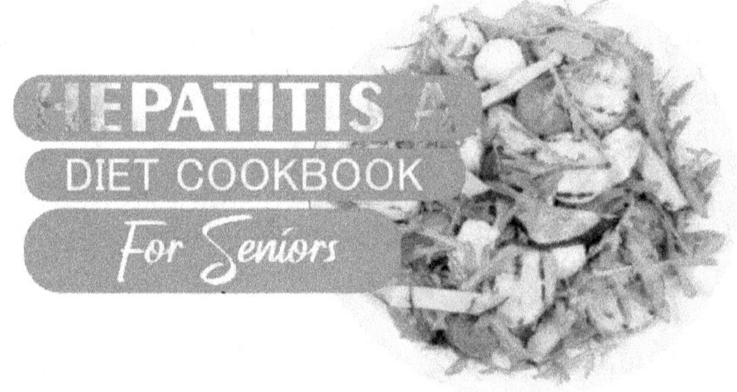

chapter 4. Dinner recipes

1. Grilled Salmon with Steamed Broccoli:

Ingredients:

- 2 salmon fillets (6 ounces each)
- 2 tablespoons olive oil
- Salt and pepper to taste 2 cups broccoli florets

Preparation:

1. Preheat grill to medium-high heat.
2. Rub salmon fillets with olive oil, then season with salt and pepper.
3. Grill salmon for 4-5 minutes on each side, or until desired doneness.
4. While salmon is grilling, steam broccoli florets for 5-7 minutes until tender.
5. Serve grilled salmon with steamed broccoli.

Nutritional Value:

- Salmon is rich in omega-3 fatty acids, protein, and micronutrients.
- Broccoli is high in fiber, vitamins C and K, and antioxidants.

Cooking Time:

Grilling salmon: 8-10 minutes Steaming broccoli: 5-7 minutes

2. Vegetable Stir-Fry

Ingredients:

- 2 cups mixed vegetables (bell peppers, carrots, snap peas, broccoli, etc.), sliced
- 2 tablespoons soy sauce
- 1 tablespoon sesame oil
- tablespoon olive oil
- cloves garlic, minced
- 1 teaspoon ginger, minced

- Salt and pepper to taste Cooked rice or noodles for serving

Preparation:

1. In a large skillet or wok, heat the olive oil on medium-high. Sauté the garlic and ginger for 1 minute.
2. Add mixed vegetables, stir-fry for 4-5 minutes until tender-crisp.
3. Drizzle with soy sauce and sesame oil, season with salt and pepper, and toss to combine.
4. Serve hot over cooked rice or noodles.

Nutritional Value:

- Mixed vegetables provide a variety of vitamins, minerals, and fiber.
- Soy sauce adds flavor with minimal calories.

Cooking Time:

Stir-frying vegetables: 4-5 minutes

Ingredients:

- 2 boneless, skinless chicken breasts
- 2 medium sweet potatoes, peeled and cubed
- 2 tablespoons olive oil
- 1 teaspoon paprika
- 1 teaspoon garlic powder
- Salt and pepper to taste Fresh parsley for garnish (optional)

Preparation:

1. Preheat oven to 400°F (200°C).
2. Place the sweet potato cubes and chicken breasts on a baking pan.
3. Drizzle with olive oil, then sprinkle with paprika, garlic powder, salt, and pepper.
4. Toss sweet potatoes to coat evenly with seasonings.
5. Bake for 25-30 minutes, or until chicken is cooked through and sweet potatoes are tender.

6. Garnish with fresh parsley if desired before serving.

Nutritional Value:

- Chicken is a good source of lean protein.
- Sweet potatoes include plenty of vitamins A and C, fiber, and antioxidants.

Cooking Time:
Baking chicken and sweet potatoes: 25-30 minutes

4. Turkey Chili

Ingredients:

- 1 pound (450g) ground turkey
- 1 tablespoon (15ml) olive oil
- 1 onion, chopped
- 3 cloves garlic, minced
- 1 bell pepper, diced
- 1 can (14 oz/400g) diced tomatoes
- 1 can (15 oz/425g) of kidney beans, drained and rinsed

- cup (240ml) chicken broth

- tablespoons (30g) chili powder

- 1 teaspoon (5g) cumin

- Salt and pepper to taste

- Optional toppings include shredded cheese, sour cream, and chopped cilantro.

Preparation:

1. In a big pot, heat olive oil over medium heat..
2. Add ground turkey and cook until browned, breaking it up with a spoon, about 5-7 minutes.
3. Add onion, garlic, and bell pepper, and cook until softened, about 5 minutes.
4. Stir in diced tomatoes, kidney beans, chicken broth, chili powder, cumin, salt, and pepper.
5. Bring to a simmer, then reduce heat to low and let simmer for 20-30 minutes. Serve hot, topped with optional toppings as desired.

Nutritional Value:

- Calories: Approximately 300 per serving (assuming 6 servings)
- Protein: Approximately 20g per serving
- Carbohydrates: Approximately 20g per serving
- Fat: Approximately 15g per serving

Cooking Time: Approximately 45 minutes

5. Pasta Primavera:

Ingredients:

- 8 oz (225g) pasta of your choice
- 2 tablespoons (30ml) olive oil
- 2 cloves garlic, minced
- 1 cup (240ml) cherry tomatoes, halved
- 1 cup (240ml) broccoli florets
- 1 cup (240ml) sliced bell peppers
- 1 cup (240ml) sliced zucchini
- Salt and pepper to taste

- Grated Parmesan cheese for serving Optional: fresh basil or parsley for garnish

Preparation:

1. Cook pasta according to package directions until al dente. Drain, then set aside.
2. In a large skillet, heat the olive oil over medium heat.
3. Add garlic and cook until fragrant, about 1 minute.
4. Add cherry tomatoes, broccoli, bell peppers, and zucchini to the skillet. Cook until vegetables are tender-crisp, about 5-7 minutes.
5. Season with salt and pepper to taste.
6. Add cooked pasta to the skillet and toss to combine.
7. Serve hot, garnished with grated Parmesan cheese and fresh herbs if desired.

Nutritional Value:
- Calories: Approximately 350 per serving (assuming 4 servings)
- Protein: Approximately 10g per serving

- Carbohydrates: Approximately 50g per serving Fat: Approximately 10g per serving

Cooking Time:
Approximately 20 minutes

6. Grilled Veggie Skewers

Ingredients:

- Assorted vegetables (such as bell peppers, zucchini, cherry tomatoes, mushrooms, onions)
- 2 tablespoons (30ml) olive oil
- 2 cloves garlic, minced
- Salt and pepper to taste Wooden or metal skewers

Preparation:

1. Preheat grill to medium-high heat.
2. Cut vegetables into bite-sized pieces.
3. In a small bowl, whisk together olive oil, garlic, salt, and pepper.

4. Thread vegetables onto skewers, alternating varieties.

5. Brush skewers with olive oil mixture.

6. Grill the skewers for 8-10 minutes, rotating regularly, until the vegetables are soft and lightly browned.

7. Serve hot as a side dish or with a dipping sauce.

Nutritional Value:

- Calories: Varies depending on vegetable selection

- Protein: Varies depending on vegetable selection

- Carbohydrates: Varies depending on vegetable selection
  Fat: Varies depending on vegetable selection

Cooking Time: Approximately 15 minutes

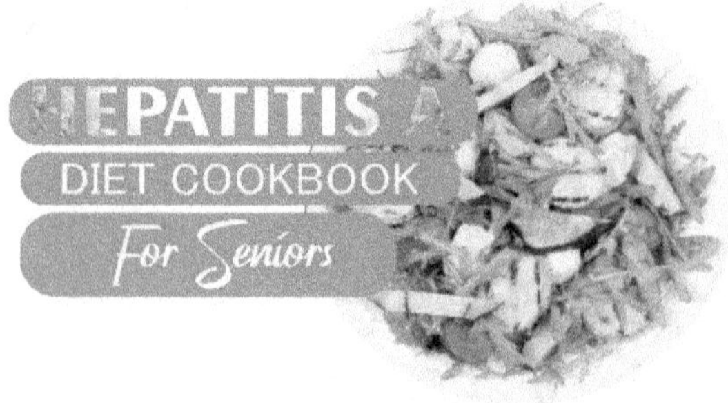

7. Lentil Soup

Ingredients:

- 1 cup dried lentils
- onion, chopped
- carrots, chopped
- celery stalks, chopped
- cloves garlic, minced
- 1 can (14 oz) diced tomatoes
- 6 cups vegetable broth
- 1 teaspoon dried thyme Salt and pepper to taste

Preparation:

1. Rinse lentils and set aside.
2. In a large pot, sauté onions, carrots, and celery until softened.
3. Add garlic and cook for another minute.
4. Stir in lentils, diced tomatoes, vegetable broth, thyme, salt, and pepper.

5. Bring to a boil, then reduce heat and simmer for about 30 minutes, or until lentils are tender.

6. Adjust seasoning if needed and serve hot.

Nutritional Value: Lentil soup is high in protein, fiber, and various vitamins and minerals such as iron, folate, and potassium.

Cooking Time: Approximately 40 minutes.

8. Baked Cod with Roasted Vegetables

Ingredients:

- 4 cod fillets (about 6 oz each)
- 2 tablespoons olive oil
- Salt and pepper to taste
- 2 bell peppers, sliced
- 1 zucchini, sliced
- onion, sliced
- cloves garlic, minced
- 1 teaspoon dried oregano

- 1 teaspoon dried thyme

Preparation:

1. Preheat oven to 400°F (200°C).
2. Place cod fillets on a baking sheet, drizzle with olive oil, and season with salt and pepper.
3. In a bowl, toss bell peppers, zucchini, onion, garlic, oregano, thyme, olive oil, salt, and pepper.
4. Arrange the vegetable mixture around the cod fillets on the baking sheet.
5. Bake for 15-20 minutes, or until the fish is cooked through and the vegetables are tender.
6. Serve hot.

Nutritional Value: Baked cod with roasted vegetables is rich in protein, omega-3 fatty acids, vitamins, and minerals.

Cooking Time: Approximately 20-25 minutes.

Ingredients:

- 4 large Portobello mushrooms
- cup quinoa
- cups vegetable broth 1 onion, diced
- 2 cloves garlic, minced
- 1 bell pepper, diced
- 1 cup spinach, chopped
- 1/4 cup grated Parmesan cheese (optional) Salt and pepper to taste

Preparation:

1. Preheat oven to 375°F (190°C).
2. Remove stems from Portobello mushrooms and scrape out the gills.
3. In a saucepan, bring vegetable broth to a boil and add quinoa. Reduce the heat, cover, and let simmer for 15-20 minutes, or until the quinoa is cooked and the liquid has been absorbed.

4. In a skillet, sauté onion, garlic, bell pepper, and spinach until softened.

5. Stir cooked quinoa into the vegetable mixture and season with salt and pepper. Spoon quinoa mixture into Portobello mushrooms and sprinkle with Parmesan cheese if desired.

6. Place the stuffed mushrooms on a baking sheet and bake for 20-25 minutes, or until soft.

7. Serve hot.

Nutritional Value: Quinoa stuffed Portobello mushrooms are a good source of protein, fiber, vitamins, and minerals.

Cooking Time: Approximately 45 minutes.

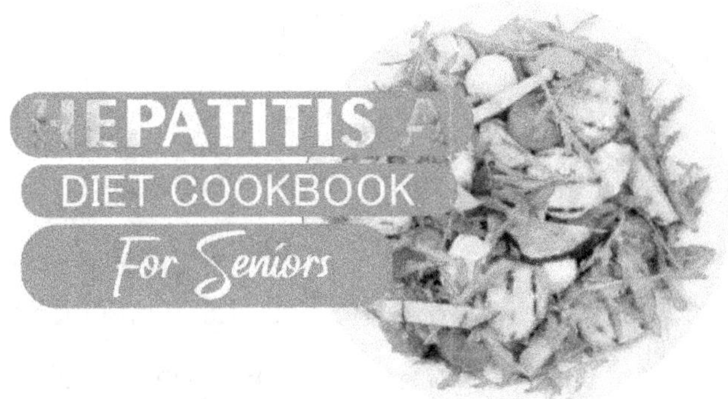

10. Vegetable Curry:

Ingredients:

- 2 tablespoons vegetable oil

- onion, diced

- cloves garlic, minced

- tablespoon grated ginger

- tablespoons curry powder

- can (14 oz) coconut milk

- cups of mixed veggies (carrots, bell peppers, broccoli, and cauliflower)

- Salt and pepper to taste

- Cooked rice or naan bread for serving

Preparation:

1. In a large skillet or saucepan, heat the vegetable oil over medium heat.

2. Add diced onion, minced garlic, and grated ginger. Sauté until fragrant. Stir in curry powder and cook for another minute.

3. Pour in coconut milk and bring to a simmer.

4. Add mixed vegetables and cook until tender, about 10-15 minutes.

5. Season with salt and pepper to taste.

6. Serve heated over cooked rice or alongside naan bread.

Nutritional Value: Vegetable curry is rich in vitamins, minerals, and healthy fats from coconut milk.

Cooking Time: Approximately 25-30 minutes.

Enjoy your cooking! If you have any further questions, feel free to ask.

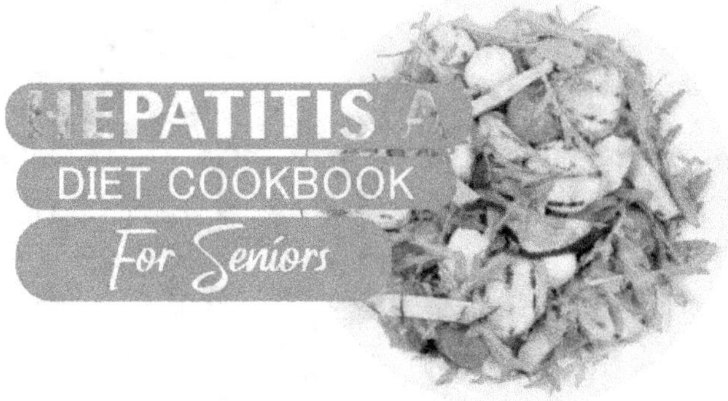

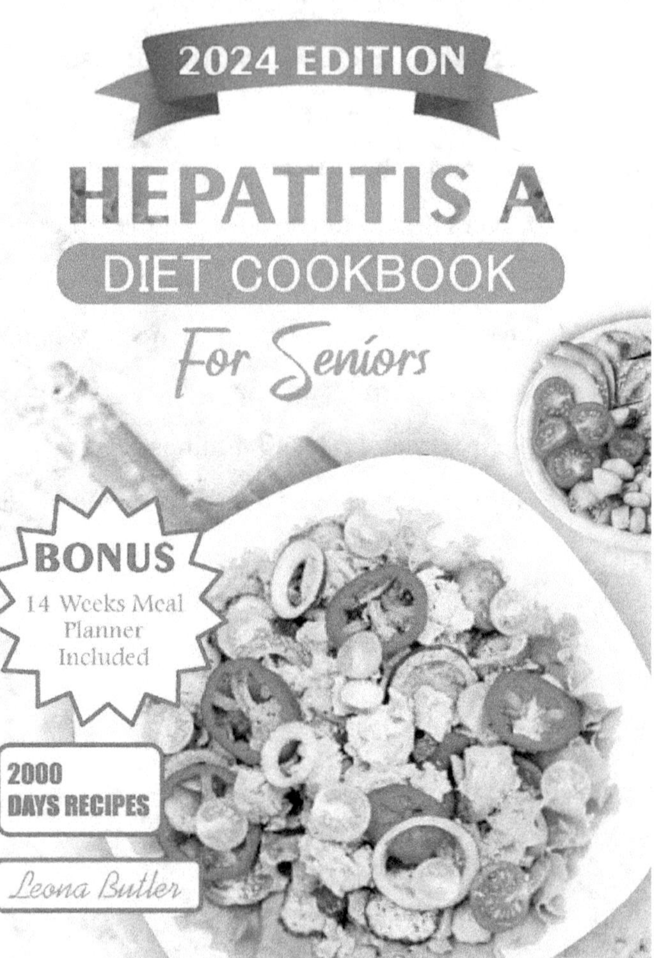

2024 EDITION
HEPATITIS A
DIET COOKBOOK
For Seniors
BONUS
14 Weeks Meal
Planner
Included
2000
DAYS RECIPES
Leona Butler

BONUS 1 : Smoothies and juicing

here are 10 smoothie and juice recipes suitable for individuals with Hepatitis A:

1. Green Cleanse Smoothie:

Ingredients:

- 1 cup spinach leaves
- 1/2 cucumber, peeled and chopped
- 1 green apple, cored and chopped
- 1/2 lemon, juiced
- 1/2 inch fresh ginger, peeled
- 1/2 cup coconut water Ice cubes (optional)

Preparation:

Wash the spinach leaves thoroughly.

In a blender, combine spinach, cucumber, apple, lemon juice, ginger, and coconut water.

Blend until smooth.

If desired, add ice cubes and re-blend.

Pour into a glass and serve immediately.

- Nutritional Value:

- Calories: 120

- Carbohydrates: 29g

- Fiber: 7g

- Protein: 3g

- Fat: 1g

- Vitamin A: 105% DV

- Vitamin C: 90% DV

- Iron: 15% DV

Cooking Time: 5 minutes

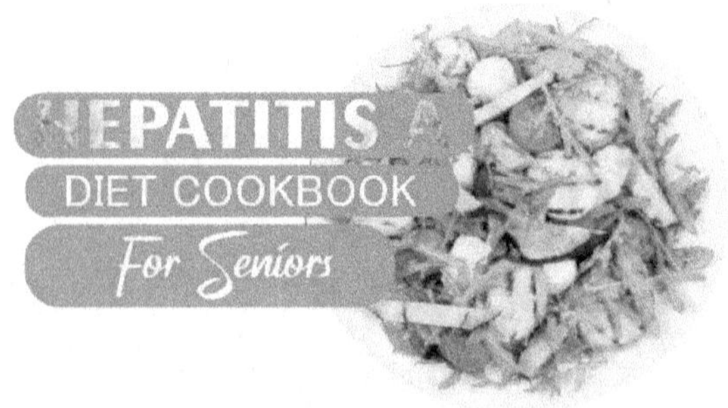

Ingredients:

- 1 cup mixed berries (such as strawberries, blueberries, and raspberries).
- 1/2 banana
- 1/2 cup Greek yogurt
- 1/2 cup almond milk 1 tablespoon honey (optional)

Preparation:

1. Wash the berries and remove any stems.
2. In a blender, combine mixed berries, banana, Greek yogurt, almond milk, and honey (if using).
3. Blend until smooth.
4. Pour into a glass and serve immediately.

Nutritional Value:

- Calories: 200
- Carbohydrates: 35g

- Fiber: 6g

- Protein: 9g

- Fat: 3g

- Vitamin C: 40% DV

- Calcium: 30% DV

- Iron: 8% DV

Cooking Time: 5 minutes

3. Citrus Delight Juice

Ingredients:

- 2 oranges, peeled and segmented

- 1 grapefruit, peeled and segmented

- 1 lime, juiced

- 1 tablespoon honey (optional) Ice cubes (optional)

Preparation:

1. Peel and segment the oranges and grapefruit.

2. In a blender, combine the orange segments, grapefruit segments, lime juice, and honey (if using).

3. Blend until smooth.

4. Add ice cubes if desired and blend again.

5. Pour into a glass and serve immediately.

Nutritional Value:

- Calories: 150

- Carbohydrates: 38g

- Fiber: 7g

- Protein: 3g

- Fat: 0g

- Vitamin C: 250% DV

- Calcium: 8% DV

- Iron: 6% DV

Cooking Time: 5 minutes

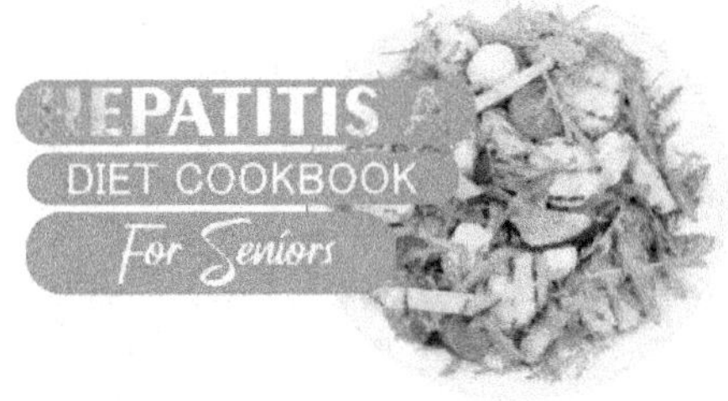

4. Liver Support Smoothie

Ingredients:

- 1 cup kale leaves, chopped
- 1/2 cup spinach leaves
- 1/2 cucumber, peeled and sliced
- 1/2 avocado, peeled and pitted
- 1/2 lemon, juiced
- 1 tablespoon fresh ginger, grated
- 1 tablespoon chia seeds 1 cup coconut water or almond milk

Preparation:

1. Combine all ingredients in a blender.
2. Blend until smooth.
3. Serve immediately.
4. Nutritional Value:
5. High in fiber, vitamins A, C, and K, and healthy fats.

Cooking Time: Prep time: 5 minutes

5. Pineapple Turmeric Cooler

Ingredients:

- 1 cup fresh pineapple chunks
- 1 small piece of fresh turmeric (about 1 inch), peeled and chopped (or 1 teaspoon turmeric powder)
- 1/2 cup coconut water
- 1 tablespoon honey or maple syrup (optional)
- Ice cubes

Preparation:

- Place all ingredients in a blender.
- Blend until smooth.
- Add more honey or maple syrup to taste, if desired.
- Serve over ice.

Cooking Time:

Prep time: 5 minutes Blend time: 2 minutes

Ingredients:

- 2 cups kale leaves, chopped
- cucumber, peeled and sliced
- green apples, cored and chopped
- 1/2 lemon, juiced
- 1 tablespoon fresh ginger, grated
- 1 tablespoon parsley, chopped
- 1 cup water or coconut water

Preparation:

1. Add all ingredients to a juicer.
2. Process until smooth.
3. Strain the juice to remove any pulp.
4. Serve immediately over ice, if desired.

Cooking Time:

Prep time: 10 minutes

Juicing time: 5 minutes

These recipes are refreshing and packed with nutrients to support your overall health and well-being. Enjoy!

Ingredients:

- 1 cup of mixed berries (such as strawberries, blueberries, raspberries)
- 1/2 cup of spinach leaves
- 1/2 cup of kale leaves
- 1/2 cup of plain Greek yogurt
- 1 tablespoon of honey
- 1/2 cup of almond milk
- 1/2 teaspoon of chia seeds Ice cubes (optional)

Preparation:

1. Wash the berries, spinach, and kale thoroughly.
2. In a blender, combine the mixed berries, spinach, kale, Greek yogurt, honey, almond milk, and chia seeds.
3. Blend until smooth.

4. If desired, add ice cubes and continue to blend until thoroughly incorporated.

5. Pour into glasses and serve immediately.

Nutritional Value:

- Provides a rich source of antioxidants, vitamins, and minerals.
- High in fiber and protein from the fruits, vegetables, and Greek yogurt.
- Low in calories and fat.

Cooking Time:

Preparation time: 5 minutes

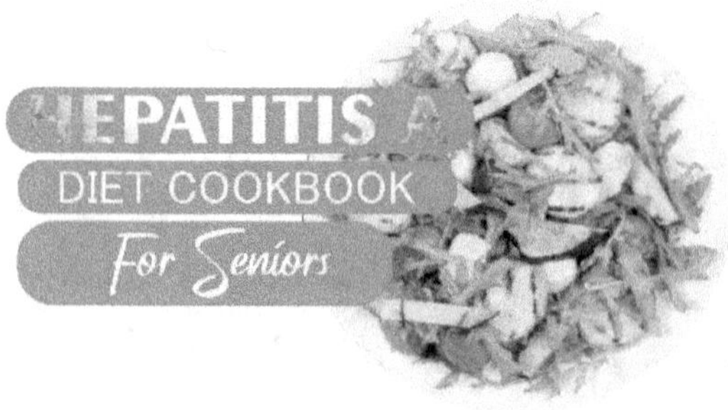

Ingredients:

- 4 large carrots, peeled and chopped
- 1-inch piece of ginger, peeled
- 1 apple, cored and chopped
- 1/2 lemon, peeled
- 1/2 cup of water

Preparation:

1. Wash and prepare all the ingredients as described.
2. In a juicer, process the carrots, ginger, apple, and lemon.
3. Add water to adjust the consistency if necessary.
4. Stir well and pour into glasses.

Preparation time: 5 minutes

9. Tropical Immunity Booster Smoothie:

Ingredients:

- 1 cup of pineapple chunks
- 1 ripe banana
- 1/2 cup of mango chunks
- 1/2 cup of orange juice
- 1/2 cup of coconut water
- 1 tablespoon of honey Ice cubes (optional)

Preparation:

1. Peel and chop the pineapple, banana, and mango.
2. In a blender, combine the pineapple, banana, mango, orange juice, coconut water, and honey.
3. Blend until smooth.
4. If desired, add ice cubes and continue to blend until thoroughly incorporated.
5. Pour into glasses and serve immediately.

Nutritional Value:

- Rich in vitamin C, vitamin A, and potassium.

- Contains natural sugars for energy boost.

- Hydrating and refreshing.

Preparation time: 5 minutes

10. Golden Beet Cleanse Juice:

Ingredients:

- 2 medium golden beets, peeled and chopped

- 2 carrots, peeled and chopped

- 1 orange, peeled and segmented

- 1-inch piece of ginger, peeled

- 1/2 lemon, peeled

- 1/2 cup of water

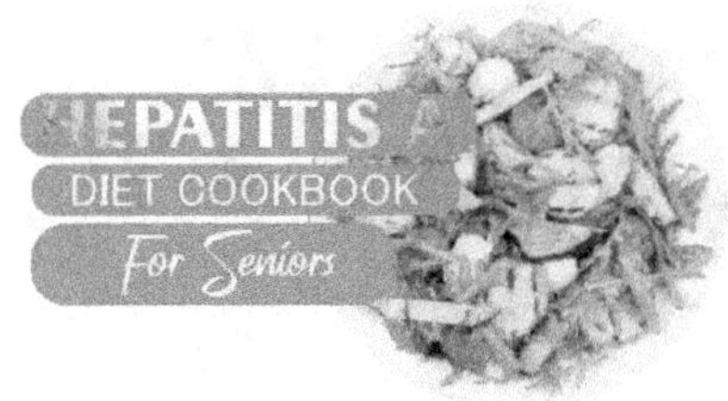

Preparation:

1. Wash, peel, and chop the golden beets, carrots, orange, and ginger.
2. In a juicer, process the golden beets, carrots, orange segments, ginger, and lemon.
3. Add water to adjust the consistency if needed.
4. Stir well and pour into glasses.

Nutritional Value:

High in antioxidants, vitamins A and C, and minerals like potassium and manganese.

Supports liver detoxification and digestion.

Cooking Time:

Preparation time: 5 minutes

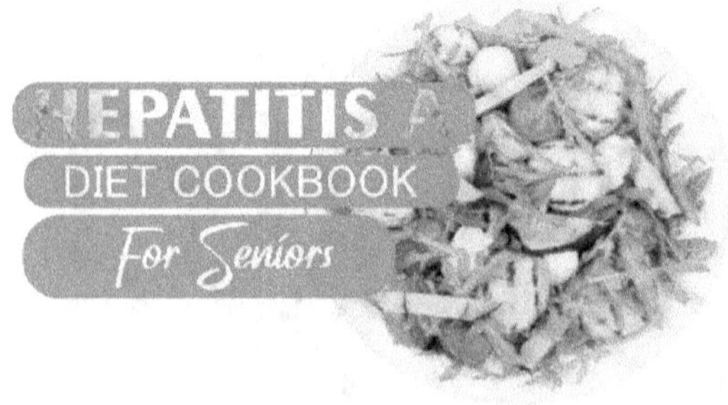

BONUS 2: 14 weeks meal planner

MY WEEKLY MEAL PLANNER

Date

	Breakfast	Lunch	Dinner
MON			
TUE			
WED			
THU			
FRI			
SAT			
SUN			

SHOPPING LIST:

-
-
-
-

TO DO LIST

NOTES AND TIPS

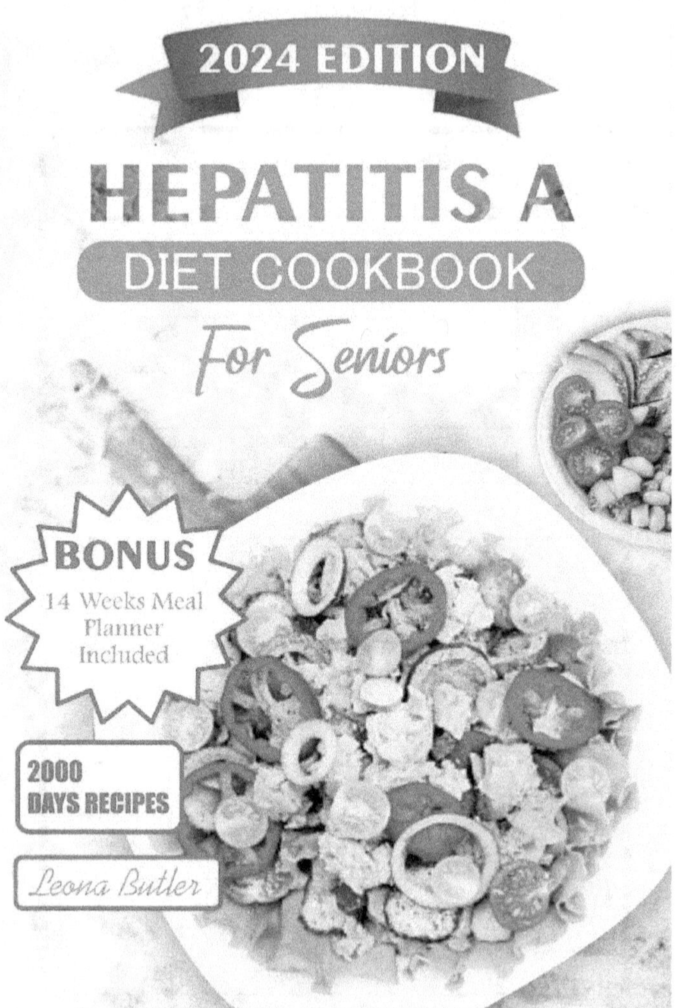

2024 EDITION

HEPATITIS A
DIET COOKBOOK
For Seniors

BONUS
14 Weeks Meal
Planner
Included

2000
DAYS RECIPES

Leona Butler

21 DAY MEAL PLAN

Day 1:

- Breakfast: Oatmeal with Blueberries
- Lunch: Grilled Chicken Salad
- Dinner: Grilled Salmon with Steamed Broccoli

Day 2:

- Breakfast: Scrambled Eggs with Spinach
- Lunch: Tuna Salad Wrap
- Dinner: Vegetable Stir-Fry

Day 3:

- Breakfast: Whole Wheat Toast with Avocado
- Lunch: Vegetable Soup
- Dinner: Baked Chicken with Roasted Sweet Potatoes

Day 4:

- Breakfast: Greek Yogurt Parfait
- Lunch: Quinoa Salad
- Dinner: Turkey Chili

Day 5:

- Breakfast: Smoothie with Spinach and Banana
- Lunch: Turkey and Avocado Sandwich
- Dinner: Pasta Primavera

Day 6:

- Breakfast: Quinoa Breakfast Bowl
- Lunch: Salmon and Asparagus
- Dinner: Grilled Veggie Skewers

Day 7:

- Breakfast: Vegetable Omelette
- Lunch: Mushroom and Spinach Quesadilla
- Dinner: Lentil Soup

Day 8:

- Breakfast: Cottage Cheese with Pineapple
- Lunch: Bean and Vegetable Wrap
- Dinner: Baked Cod with Roasted Vegetables

Day 9:

- Breakfast: Whole Grain Pancakes
- Lunch: Egg Salad Lettuce Wraps
- Dinner: Quinoa Stuffed Bell Peppers

Day 10:

- Breakfast: Egg and Veggie Muffins
- Lunch: Quinoa Stuffed Portobello Mushrooms
- Dinner: Vegetable Curry

Day 11:

- Breakfast: Oatmeal with Blueberries
- Lunch: Grilled Chicken Salad
- Dinner: Grilled Salmon with Steamed Broccoli

Day 12:

- Breakfast: Scrambled Eggs with Spinach
- Lunch: Tuna Salad Wrap
- Dinner: Vegetable Stir-Fry

Day 13:

- Breakfast: Whole Wheat Toast with Avocado
- Lunch: Vegetable Soup
- Dinner: Baked Chicken with Roasted Sweet Potatoes

Day 14:

- Breakfast: Greek Yogurt Parfait
- Lunch: Quinoa Salad
- Dinner: Turkey Chili

Day 15:

- Breakfast: Smoothie with Spinach and Banana
- Lunch: Turkey and Avocado Sandwich
- Dinner: Pasta Primavera

Day 16:

- Breakfast: Quinoa Breakfast Bowl

- Lunch: Salmon and Asparagus

- Dinner: Grilled Veggie Skewers

Day 17:

- Breakfast: Vegetable Omelette

- Lunch: Mushroom and Spinach Quesadilla

- Dinner: Lentil Soup

Day 18:

- Breakfast: Cottage Cheese with Pineapple

- Lunch: Bean and Vegetable Wrap

- Dinner: Baked Cod with Roasted Vegetables

Day 19:

- Breakfast: Whole Grain Pancakes

- Lunch: Egg Salad Lettuce Wraps

- Dinner: Quinoa Stuffed Bell Peppers

Day 20:

- Breakfast: Egg and Veggie Muffins

- Lunch: Quinoa Stuffed Portobello Mushrooms

- Dinner: Vegetable Curry

Day 21:

- Breakfast: Oatmeal with Blueberries

- Lunch: Grilled Chicken Salad

- Dinner: Grilled Salmon with Steamed Broccoli

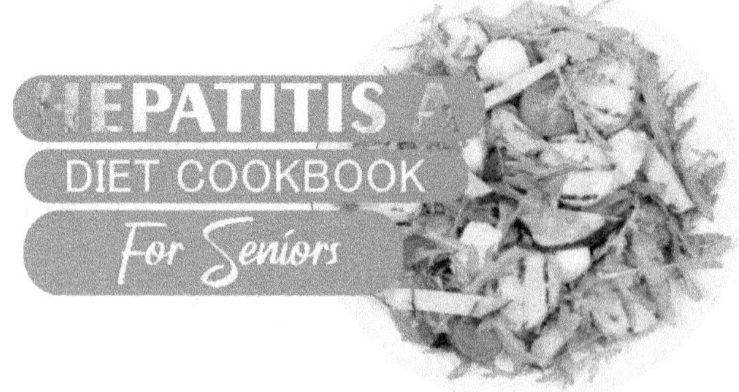

Conclusion

In conclusion, the Hepatitis A Diet Cookbook for Seniors not only offers delicious and nutritious recipes tailored to support individuals battling Hepatitis A, but it also serves as a beacon of hope and empowerment for seniors navigating this health challenge. By providing comprehensive dietary guidance, practical tips, and flavorful meal ideas, this cookbook not only promotes physical well-being but also enhances the overall quality of life for seniors affected by Hepatitis A.

Through the power of food, it fosters a sense of control and agency, empowering seniors to actively manage their health and embrace a fulfilling lifestyle. As we close this chapter, let us remember that a nourishing diet is not just about sustenance; it is a form of self-care and resilience. May this cookbook continue to inspire seniors on their journey to wellness and serve as a testament to the healing potential of wholesome, delicious meals.

Thank you for taking the time to explore the Hepatitis A Diet Cookbook For Seniors. Your interest in supporting senior health is truly appreciated. By engaging with this cookbook, you're not only enriching your own knowledge but also potentially improving the lives of seniors facing health challenges.

Your commitment to understanding dietary needs and advocating for healthier lifestyles for seniors is commendable. Every page turned and recipe considered is a step towards empowering seniors to lead fulfilling lives despite health obstacles.

Your support in spreading awareness about hepatitis A and promoting nutritious eating habits among seniors is invaluable. Together, we can make a difference in the lives of our elderly community members. Thank you for being a part of this journey towards better health and well-being for seniors.

MY WEEKLY MEAL PLANNER

Date

	Breakfast	Lunch	Dinner
MON			
TUE			
WED			
THU			
FRI			
SAT			
SUN			

SHOPPING LIST:

-
-
-
-

To Do List

NOTES AND TIPS

MY WEEKLY MEAL PLANNER

Date

	Breakfast	Lunch	Dinner
MON			
TUE			
WED			
THU			
FRI			
SAT			
SUN			

SHOPPING LIST:

-
-
-
-

TO DO LIST

NOTES AND TIPS

MY WEEKLY MEAL PLANNER

Date

	Breakfast	Lunch	Dinner
MON			
TUE			
WED			
THU			
FRI			
SAT			
SUN			

SHOPPING LIST:

-
-
-
-

To Do List

NOTES
AND TIPS

MY WEEKLY MEAL PLANNER

Date

	Breakfast	Lunch	Dinner
MON			
TUE			
WED			
THU			
FRI			
SAT			
SUN			

SHOPPING LIST:

To Do List

NOTES
AND TIPS

MY WEEKLY MEAL PLANNER

Date

	Breakfast	Lunch	Dinner
MON			
TUE			
WED			
THU			
FRI			
SAT			
SUN			

SHOPPING LIST:

- ● ....
- ● ....
- ● ....
- ● ....

TO DO LIST

....
....
....
....
....

NOTES
AND TIPS

MY WEEKLY MEAL PLANNER

Date

	Breakfast	Lunch	Dinner
MON			
TUE			
WED			
THU			
FRI			
SAT			
SUN			

SHOPPING LIST:

To Do List

NOTES
AND TIPS

MY WEEKLY MEAL PLANNER

Date

	Breakfast	Lunch	Dinner
MON			
TUE			
WED			
THU			
FRI			
SAT			
SUN			

SHOPPING LIST:

-
-
-
-

TO DO LIST

NOTES AND TIPS

MY WEEKLY MEAL PLANNER

Date

	Breakfast	Lunch	Dinner
MON			
TUE			
WED			
THU			
FRI			
SAT			
SUN			

SHOPPING LIST:

To Do List

NOTES
AND TIPS

MY WEEKLY MEAL PLANNER

Date

	Breakfast	Lunch	Dinner
MON			
TUE			
WED			
THU			
FRI			
SAT			
SUN			

SHOPPING LIST:

To Do List

- ● . . . .
- ● . . . .
- ● . . . .
- ● . . . .

NOTES
AND TIPS

MY WEEKLY MEAL PLANNER

Date

	Breakfast	Lunch	Dinner
MON			
TUE			
WED			
THU			
FRI			
SAT			
SUN			

SHOPPING LIST:

To Do List

NOTES AND TIPS

MY WEEKLY MEAL PLANNER

Date

	Breakfast	Lunch	Dinner
MON			
TUE			
WED			
THU			
FRI			
SAT			
SUN			

SHOPPING LIST:

To Do List

NOTES AND TIPS

MY WEEKLY MEAL PLANNER

Date

	Breakfast	Lunch	Dinner
MON			
TUE			
WED			
THU			
FRI			
SAT			
SUN			

SHOPPING LIST:

- ....
- ....
- ....
- ....

TO DO LIST

....
....
....
....

NOTES
AND TIPS

MY WEEKLY MEAL PLANNER

Date

	Breakfast	Lunch	Dinner
MON			
TUE			
WED			
THU			
FRI			
SAT			
SUN			

SHOPPING LIST:

-
-
-
-

TO DO LIST

NOTES AND TIPS

MY WEEKLY MEAL PLANNER

Date

	Breakfast	Lunch	Dinner
MON			
TUE			
WED			
THU			
FRI			
SAT			
SUN			

SHOPPING LIST:

To Do List

NOTES
AND TIPS